WEIGHT LOSS HABITS

AMINE SALHI

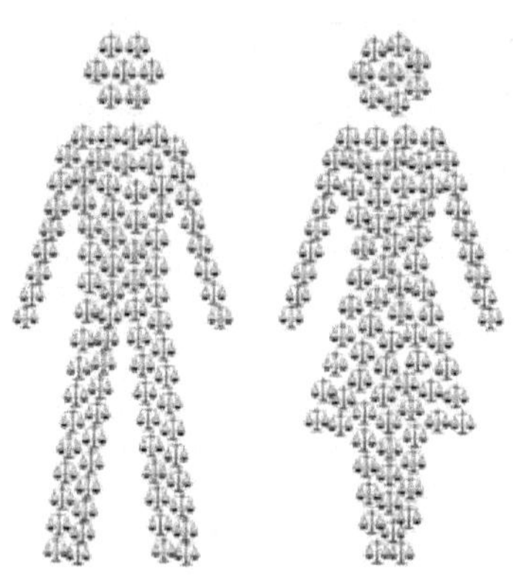

This e-book is offered as an overview of the fad diets that are taking over the internet and clouding the reality of the body's need for a balance between diet and exercise to achieve healthy weight loss and overall good health.

Author

Table of Contents

CHAPTER ONE

WHAT IS A FAD? (AND WHY YOUR BODY IS NOT ONE)

I would like to begin this chapter by introducing myself. I am you. I mean, quite obvious I am not but I am a general consumer of internet knowledge in the pursuit of becoming my best self despite the realization that so much of the knowledge that is presented in the present will not be relevant by the time I sit down to write this page. In other words, the information, or at least what is considered current and relevant, changes so rapidly that the access date is not necessary to create some form of valid citation to a document. We must literally state, "well, that is what it said yesterday," to validate our claims. Yet, of course, we trust everything online regardless of when it was published or who decided that it was relevant to our search criteria. We believe, with few exceptions, what the media tells us to be true. We believe, with few exceptions, what the media tells us that we should be. We even believe, with few exceptions, who the media tells us that we should be. Who am I? I am you. I am stuck in this vertex between who I know I am and who I am told that I should be. Of course, I have one advantage. I am painfully aware of where I am. I know that the fads of the modern society dictate my interactions. My fear is that these very fads are creating health disparities that my not fully manifest until the limitations on access to health care are so significant that those who suffer from these fads are no longer eligible for care.

When I decided to write a book about healthy weight loss, the first thing that I did was try to get a baseline understanding about what you, the reader, have accessed through popular media and the internet. I looked to find what was popular and how it is being presented to information consumers around the world. Popular! That was the keyword that stuck in my mind. So often, we believe that in order to be popular, we must follow what it is popular. We must identify with the same plights that the media represents and adhere to the trends of the majority in order to keep from being left behind in the dark ages. But guess what… What is popular today will almost certainly not be popular tomorrow. What is trending today will be yesterday's news in a just a few short clicks. What is popular is, without the benefit of another word, nothing more than a fad.

There is that word, again, that seems to engulf the data on weight loss strategies and nearly every trend that can be found online. But what does it mean and why are fads so bad? On the surface, fads are not bad but rather they are something that gains a great deal of active interest gaining rapid popularity that lasts only a short period and then quickly give way to another interest or trend. There is no way to suggest that fads are either good or bad nor to debate their relevance in society. Fads are found in every market and often define a generation or at least mark many laughable moments once the fad has passed. The negative reminders, whether photographs online of last year's fashion fads or long term medical issues, remain, but the interest and popularity fade away leaving questions as to how so many people once accepted this interest as the norm or a symbol of popularity. In this sense, a fad can be defined as something that is quickly accepted but its popularity is short lived leaving behind only negative reminders of its otherwise forgotten presence.

As this is not a book on sociology, I turn now to how this applies to your weight loss journey and why I ask that you not consider this journey as a fad. Given the definition of a fad, let's put into perspective what you are trying to achieve. Quite obviously, as your search brought you to a book on healthy weight loss, your interests is not in a quick fix but rather on a sustainable lifestyle change that can promote health and longevity. Your interests are not focused on the popularity of the journey but rather on the outcomes. Popularity refers to someone or something that is given a high value. I assume, as you are here, that you place a high value in yourself or, at the very least, are working towards the assignment of this value. Therefore, you are already popular to who matters most and, if it counts, I value you as well. Therefore, being popular is not what makes a fad concerning. Instead, I want you to turn your attention to the concept of being short lived. While I can understand that you might want for this journey to be one and done, I can assure you that a short lived weight loss journey yields short lived results. Your journey to health is represented by your journey for longevity. Is short lived how you would define this journey?

This leads to the book's title and my primary purpose for writing. Just as your journey can not be viewed as short term, your pursuit of a healthy weight should be reflective of your pursuit of a long and healthy life. Your body is not a fad. The goal should not be to have the media represented perfect body for a short period and then to fade away. The weight loss journey should not end abruptly leaving nothing enduring except for the negative health implications and the psychological turmoil associated with the weight returning. If your goal is to have a sustainable body, then you must have a sustainable weight loss journey. If your goal is to achieve a healthy weight so that you can enjoy the best life possible, pursue other interests, and feel a true sense of value in yourself, then you can no longer treat your body as if it is a fad. You must, instead, make a commitment to your body that you will go the distance and integrate sustainable diet and exercise changes that may not give the immediate popular results but rather will ensure that once these results are achieved, they will be sustained.

In the following chapters I will present to you the concept of fad diets along with the pros and cons of many popular fad diets that I am certain you have come across. Although these will be presented, I would like to add that I, in no way, endorse any fad diets. I would also like to suggest that you speak with your healthcare professional before beginning any weight loss strategy. Yet, I feel the need to include these as a failure to acknowledge the information available would be dismissive of your personal search for what will work. I understand the appeal of fad diets but, as I stated, I value you and would love nothing more than to promote your longevity over your immediate results. After the general overview of these fad diets, I will then direct your attention to what is sustainable, based in evidence, and certain to ensure a healthy weight loss and improved overall health. After all, if longevity and health do not go hand in hand, being healthy would be nothing more than a fad.

CHAPTER TWO

WHAT IS A FAD DIET?

As we have already discussed what a fad is and how it should not be applied to your definition of your body or your weight loss journey, it is now important that we establish the context of the term in the over saturated world of diet strategies. Fad diets can be discussed in two applications. The first of these is through the concept of popularity. These diets are popular for a short period in the media and then quickly fade away. However, what is most often the case is that the popularity of the diets remains high regardless of any of the other implications. Instead, the popularity of the diet for the individual fades making the diet unsustainable. The second notion is that the outcomes or results of the diets are short lived once the popularity fades away. In fact, in many instances, the results are countered with an increased weight gain upon return to normal food consumption.

Yet, let's say that you are completely committed to weight loss and have every bit of determination to sustain the fad diet as the immediate results outweigh the concerns and the risk of additional weight gain is not relevant to you as you will not return to previous dietary habits. I remember many fads as an adolescent that my mother told me would fade and I swore that I would never regret. I was committed! Fortunately, permanent hair dye is not really permanent and I have since learned the true meaning of commitment. The fact is, that these diets cannot sustain your body's needs and therefore are not sustainable. Why? Quite simply fad diets require that you limit or eliminate at least one essential food group creating a deficit in your dietary intake of vitamins and nutrients essential for health and longevity. Without such intake, your body will respond in the immediate with a rapid weight loss. However, this does not mean that your body is rewarding your for depriving it of essential fuel for longevity but rather that your body is letting you know that something is wrong. The body does not know popularity, media portrayal of the perfect image, or your personal reasons for wanting to lose weight. The body does not understand why you are depriving it when your interdependency is so blatantly obvious. Eventually, your body will demand nutrition or respond through illness and an overall sense of unhealthiness.

If these diets lead to unhealthiness and are not sustainable, then why are they so popular? Certainly, every person who promotes weight loss through the use of fad diets is not trying to cause all those who listen to suffer these negative outcomes. We've all read the claims that these secrets are known to doctors but kept away from the public for various reasons ranging from contradicting research to conspiracies involving the pharmaceutical companies. I can assure you that medical professionals take an oath to put the public's health as their priority. If there was a secret strategy to achieve rapid weight loss, ending the risk factor of obesity associated with diabetes, cardiovascular disease, and high mortality rates, medical professionals would jump at the opportunity to share this secret with their patients. You would never see an overweight medical professional and no relative of these professionals would struggle with their weight. If there was such a secret, then it would be shared. The fact is that the desire for rapid weight loss is fulfilled through these fad diets and only these "success stories" are highlighted in the media. In other words, only what is popular is communicated while the truthfulness of the negative implications remains hidden behind the currency of the fad.

To clarify, fad diets are simply fads that are represented by what is popular (rapid weight loss) but these results are not sustainable as they interfere with the body's needs and your relationship with your body. This relationship, the one between your inner self and your body, determines your own mortality. This relationship determines your own sustainability. Regardless of your commitment to weight loss, your commitment to your body should be of far greater interest to you than what is popular in the media. A fad diet is not only unstainable, but the results and your health will also suffer the same fate.

Despite my obvious distrust of fad diets, I want to ensure you that I am biased through fairness. In other words, these assertions are not vaguely based in what I have been taught to suggest but rather come through extensive research into the supposed science that supports the use of these diets, an acknowledgement of their often efficacy in rapid weight loss, and my knowledge of the nutritional needs for a healthy body. Therefore, the following brief chapter will provide an overview of the claims for each fad diet, the general guidelines, and the concerns associated with nutritional deficiencies. In no way should this be taken as a guide for implementing any of these diets but rather serves as a way to show the importance of balance while answer general questions about the fad diets readily available on the internet.

CHAPTER THREE

THE KETOGENIC DIET

I begin with the popular keto (ketogenic) diet as it has taken the diet and weight loss literature by a strong hold. Commonly coupled with the Atkins diet in terms of discussion, the keto diet differs significantly in the science. There is little to no debate that cutting out nearly all carbohydrates will result in weight loss. However, the keto diet, which was originally and successfully developed to treat epilepsy, focuses on high fat intake, moderate protein intake, and ideally less than 5% carbohydrate intake per day. According to the research presented by Ellenbroek, et al. (2014) the body responds to the lack of glucose which is found in the carbohydrates and proteins, by becoming fat adapted or entering ketosis. During this state, the body does not use glucose for fuel but rather the liver produces ketones which serve to fuel the body. The idea is that the body will be able to burn the fat present causing a reduced appetite.

The initial weight loss is water weight as carbohydrates require hydration. As this is not longer needed, there is a nearly immediate drop in weight often referred to as a flush. The body then undergoes a serious of changes that are necessary to support the use of fat for fuel and reduce the dependency on glucose. This can result in what is commonly referred to as the keto flu in which the dieter becomes fatigued, suffers from extreme headaches, stomach irritability, and restlessness. If the dieter is able to manage through the keto flu, then they have successfully found themselves in ketosis and their body no longer craves glucose. Of course, this does not mean that you will not want glucose nor that the body has accepted this new arrangement. In fact, as dehydration is a serious concern (you did not think all of that water was there for no reason, did you) then you must also consider all of the implications of dehydration. Keto enthusiasts recommend a wide range of nutritional supplements but focus primarily on the use of supplemental electrolytes, added salt intake, and increased fat consumption.

There are two significant areas of concern that I would like to point out. Firstly, if your body no longer uses glucose for fuel, what happens to that one piece of cake at your cousin's wedding that it would be simply too rude to decline? What does you body do when you decide that you just want to eat an apple a day because your digestive track is suffering? Surely corn or beans could not mean the end of ketosis and the realization that you must now go back through the keto flu to stay on track! According to Ellenbroek, et al. (2014) the second area of concern is what we do not know about the long term effects of using the keto diet for weight loss. Although the diet is not new, the general use of it for weight loss has only recently become popular. Prior to this, the only research focused on the cost to benefit analysis when considering patients with epilepsy. Yet, in a recent study, Ellenbroek, et al. (2014) found no long term weight loss but rather insulin resistance in mice and further suggested an increased risk in kidney complications and osteoporosis. Yet, in the short term, the quick weight loss should justify the unknown, right?

In brief, the keto diet was never intended for weight loss and the effects of its long term use, despite the obvious difficulties in sustaining this diet, are yet unknown. The immediate weight loss is the result of dehydration which then requires an extensive array of supplements rather than simply consuming nutrient rich foods in moderation. The keto diet increases the amount of fat consumed, despite concerns ranging from high cholesterol to high blood pressure, and reduces the number of carbohydrates to a point so low as to require the body to forego the natural process of burning glucose to fuel the body systems.

Chapter Four

The Atkins Diet

The Atkins diet is not nearly as new to the scene of fad diets and is often referred to as a relative of the ketogenic diet. Notably, both diets restrict the intake of carbohydrates and, according to the Atkins website, the diet is essentially a keto diet in that it restricts carbohydrates in an order to reach a state of ketosis in which the body burns fat instead of glucose. However, the difference is in the proportion of fat to protein in the guidelines. The Atkins website explains that the Atkins diet is more flexible allowing 20-30% daily intake of protein and up to 15% carbohydrate. The Atkins diet does not call for as many restrictions and therefore allows for some intake of essential nutrients. However, the fact remains that, no matter how many different boxes are labeled as Atkins in the supermarket, the restriction of essential nutrients brings to question the sustainability of the diet and the body's long term response to these changes.

It is important to note that, as the Atkins diet also restricts carbohydrates to the point of achieving ketosis and becoming a fat burner, even though it is less restrictive, there are serious dangers associated with this process. Not only are the same concerns relating to dehydration and the need for supplements significant, but researcher Mamounis (2017) has found that this process can cause irreversible damage enzyme and hormone regulation as well as lead to insulin resistance. The science, however, is limited according to Mamounis (2017) as what is currently considered longitudinal research studies consist of generally no more than one year meaning that, despite the fact that the Atkins diet has been circulating for decades, no actual long term emphasis on the effects has been conducted. Why, you may ask. Quite simply, this is a fad diet that is given little merit in the research as it is not anticipated that most people will be able to sustain the diet for a longer period. Therefore, studying the effects beyond the year point seems relatively moot. No matter how committed you are, there is not enough data to suggest that this is a safe avenue for long term weight management and certainly not enough to justify any long term negative effects to your health. Instead, I ask that you be diligent in looking beyond the marketing techniques and consider the science, or lack thereof, for the long term sustainability of this fad diet.

CHAPTER FIVE

THE JUICE DIET

Of course, some fad diets are so blatantly intended to be short lived that the very concept of the diet is based in brevity. Here, I speak of the juice diet which is also referred to as the juice detox or cleanse. The concept of the juice diet is to cleanse the body through abstaining from solid foods and only intaking the nutrient richness of fruit and vegetable juices. Of course, many of the nutrients found in fruits and vegetables, such as fiber, are not found in the sweet juices but rather in the pulp and skin of the produce. Clearly, it may be possible to lose a few pounds over the 3 days to 1 week that you suffer through this diet, but there is no lifestyle change, the body does not receive what it needs, and the body will rapidly hold to any nutrients that it receives once normal eating resumes. In other words, whatever you lose during this period will likely be met with additional weight following the experience. I am not sure about you, but I do not see the benefits to this experience given the lack of evidence that supports any nutritional or long term gains from the juice diet.

However, in the spirit of fairness, I have spent some time researching the science or pseudoscience behind this fad diet in hopes to give you a brief overview and prevent you from spending countless hours trying to uncover some hidden truths that may be present. Three pages into Google Scholar, using both the search terms of juice diet for weight loss and juice diet detox, yielded no peer reviewed studies. Instead, several opinion articles were found. Finally, on the fifth page, I found an article presented by Heaner (2013). The article began by explaining that detoxification diets such as juicing are not only appealing to dieters but rather to all types of people who are concerned about the amount of toxins to which they are exposed through the environment and their diet. I was intrigued assuming that this meant that there was some truth to the fad and yet also slightly wondering if I had missed something.

Of course, the example provided was of a woman who lost approximately 10 pounds after the juice cleanse but then found herself 20 pounds heavier not long after returning to her normal dietary consumption. Why? It is simple, when we deprive our body of key nutrients for an extended period, even as brief as a week, the body responds by trying to hold onto these nutrients and any excess once normal consumption is restored. Not only is the weight lost regained, but this means that the body fights back by storing even more! How is that for a good relationship? Yet, the article mentioned detoxification and, like you, I have often wondered if getting rid of these contaminants might free up my body to focus on normal metabolic functions. But, guess what! That's right, there is no scientific evidence to suggest that the juice diet, or any diet for that matter, detoxifies the body. Instead, Heaner (2013) explained that detoxifying is a medical term used when a patient has a build up of heavy metals or has experienced substance abuse and is undergoing withdrawal. However, even in these extreme cases, the juice diet is not on the list of interventions.

In brief, the juice diet is a way to lose a quick amount of weight for the purpose of stating that you lost a quick amount of weight. Of course, this statement will only be relevant for a short period as you will then have to explain the rapid weight gain and begin the next course of yo-yo dieting. I feel safe in stating that neither of us want that for you. I also hope that I can assume that if you are in need of medical detoxification that you will seek medical attention rather than attempting a fad diet that will be of no medical use for you. Based on these claims and assumptions, I can confidently state that the juice diet is a fad diet that we can move on from.

Chapter Six

Intermittent Fasting

If limiting a certain food group for the purpose of weight loss can have significant negative implications for one's health, then perhaps the answer is to limit overall intake during certain periods to allow the body to "catch up" to the amount of intake that has been stored. This is the concept behind intermittent fasting. According to Bryant (2017) intermittent fasting is often considered a religious practice meaning that there are some indications that the practice could be good for the soul. It is okay. You can read that last statement again (I had to). As I have repeatedly stated that there must be a balance between mind, body, and spirit, perhaps this fad diet is onto something. However, also recall that I stated that we must not give up the needs of one to support the other as this could lead to a serious imbalance. Therefore, we must research a bit more into the effects of intermittent fasting. According to Bryant (2017) the fad is more than related to religiosity but rather based in the idea that seriously restricting caloric intake on certain days to create a cycle will signal the body to burn what it already has stored. For some, this cycle is based on the number of days of normal consumption while others fast for extended period per day allowing themselves only set hours in which they can consume foods.

Now, let's get to the important questions. Does it work and is it sustainable? According to Bryant (2017) there is limited evidence to support the use of this strategy for weight loss showing that there is little to no difference between standard weight loss strategies and intermittent fasting. There have been studies, however, to show unstable glucose levels, stiffness in the heart muscles, and excessive consumption on days or time periods were not in effect. In other words, while the body was supposed to catch up during fasting, the intake was caught up during periods of consumption. This means that there are obvious negative health risks while there remains little to no evidence that supports this fad diet. Additionally, let's not forget the discomfort of being hungry for either days at a time or the majority of the hours in a day. I do not think that this lifestyle, even if the data was stronger, would be sustainable for myself or for others who are looking for a way to achieve overall health and healthy weight loss. After all, I do not know about you but the feeling of being "hangry" certainly does not do justice for my mind or spirit but can cause serious complications in my relationships with others. In other words, I believe that this practice should be left to the religious traditions while the nutritional guidance should focus on physical health.

CHAPTER SEVEN

THE VEGETARIAN DIET

As we have discussed a variety of lifestyle and quick fix diets that highly controversial and offer little to no scientific justification for putting your body through these deficits, I now turn to a more sustainable lifestyle data and do so with the understanding that many people have moral and religious reasons for following this diet. I also have extensive knowledge as to the alternative sources of nutrients that are utilized in the vegetarian diet so I must disclaim that I do not consider this so much a fad diet but rather an alternative diet that, when not properly followed or followed for reasons of popularity, can lead to serious negative health outcomes. Just as the following section includes a discussion of eating disorders, I believe that a true conversation about health eating and weight loss must not steer clear of topics that may be debatable as this would lead to a one sided communication. Personally, I rarely enjoy conversating with myself and would by far prefer gaining a true understanding of others through these topics. Yet, I recall a friend of mine "going vegetarian" because his significant other had chosen this lifestyle. When I had asked her about her decision, she said that it began in high school as a form of rebellion to her stepmother's cooking and just stuck. Later, she tried to eat meat again and found her that her body "rejected it" fiercely. Perhaps it was this friend's choice to follow that has led me to include vegetarianism as a fad diet or perhaps it is simply because there are concerns about the proper nutritional intakes of proteins and healthy fats for those on this diet. Regardless, it differs from the concept of a balanced diet that is the focus of this book and therefore, you deserve an overview of the benefits and risks associated.

Again, in the effort to be fair and the acknowledgement that I have my own experiences and perceptions of vegetarianism, I turn to the current research about the eating lifestyle. According to Pilis, Stec, Zych, and Pilis (2014) vegetarianism is strictly the avoidance of eating meat products that can stem from economical, ecological, religious, health, or ethical considerations. The researchers further noted that, no matter why a person adopts this way of eating, when properly implemented, they will lose weight and achieve a greater balance between carbohydrate intake and the intake of high fat foods. In other words, the vegetarian diet is more carbohydrate based than protein and fat. As I have asserted obvious concerns about diets that suppress the intake of carbohydrates, one would assume that I would quickly recommend the opposite approach. Of course, one would be wrong. The body has very specific needs which have been expressed in countless research studies and the negative implications of restrictions have been clearly identified in these studies. For vegetarianism, cardiovascular disorders and limitations on metabolic and endocrine functions are highly documented. Furthermore, women have experienced menstrual dysfunction and there have been countless studies to support the concern for protein deficiencies. In other words, the opposite side of the spectrum does not achieve a balance but is simply on the opposite side of the middle.

Vegetarianism is, to some extent, sustainable as there are many alternatives to meats that have been made readily available. Fat and protein can be integrated into the diet through alternative products making it possible to achieve a balanced dietary intake without consuming meat. However, given the various reasons, including economic, that people choose this lifestyle, one must also consider the costs of these alternatives. Do all vegetarians achieve an actual balance of nutrients? Is there enough knowledge about these alternatives and their availability to support this diet as a common choice or should it remain on the list of fad diets? Certainly, these are not questions that can be answered here, today. However, they are important considerations if this is an option that you are currently investigating for your weight loss journey. The key, here, is to investigate. How much access do you have to alternative protein and healthy fat sources? Is weight loss your only reason for considering vegetarianism? If so, remember that returning to a typical diet is not as easy as going to the supermarket. Most importantly, would you be considering this option if there was a simpler way to achieving a healthy weight loss and overall health? If not, stay with me a bit longer. We just might find your answer!

Chapter Eight

Eating Disorders

Although the emphasis of the current book is on healthy weight loss over the use of dangerous fad diets, there is also a truthfulness as to how the media influences our food consumption decisions, body image, and desire to fit a certain profile. For many, this results in failed attempts at fad diets or a collection of information gathered with little focus on applying the knowledge to true lifestyle changes. However, for some, these attempts at fad diets and emphasis on the media portrayals can trigger psychological responses that lead to eating disorders. I feel compelled to provide a general overview as to these processes as achieving health through weight loss must include whole health. In other words, just as we depend on our body for sustainability, our body depends on our mind and spirit. In order to achieve whole health, we must not neglect one to improve the other.

According to Khawandanah and Tewfik (2016) there is a difference between a desire to lose weight through fad diets and eating disorders but it is not possible to miss the clear relationship between the two. The researchers explain that fad diets often promise the quickest way to achieve the ideal image as portrayed in the media. However, when these diets are not sustainable, the dieters may feel as if they have failed or something is wrong with their body. Adding this to the already distorted body image, Khawandanah and Tewfik (2016) explained that the individual can experience the negative physical and psychological consequences of yo-yo dieting which can include heart disease, cancer, and an imbalance of the stress hormone cortisol. The extreme highs and lows associated with weight loss and weight gain can then lead to an unhealthy relationship with food and nutrition. Khawandanah and Tewfik (2016) added that the two most frequently associated eating disorders are anorexia nervosa and bulimia. The former of these is characterized by a complete aversion to food in which the individual consumes only the minimal necessary to avoid detection of the disorder. In the latter, the practice of binging and purging through either vomiting or the use of laxatives is justified by the distorted body image. In both, a history of a complex relationship with food and poor self-image can typically be identified.

Although you have found yourself here, in the fourth chapter of this book, due to a search for a healthy way to lose weight and maintain a healthy balance, the potential for these negative outcomes are there for anyone who struggles with weight loss and has looked towards or attempted fad diets. Fortunately, the science in the psychological field of dieting has far surpassed that of fad diets which means that there is help available. The media is a powerful tool and we all fall prey to the promises on occasions. The important emphasis must remain on overall health and the prevention of negative outcomes associated with quick responses to the media portrayal of the popular image. When there is an imbalance in this emphasis, it is essential that the help to overcome these challenges be sought and health restored. As I speak frequently on a healthy weight loss to achieve overall health, I ask that you consider your own personal circumstances and consult with your physician to determine a healthy weight goal for your body type. My purpose is not to provide a strict guideline for weight loss or provide a specific image that you should aim to achieve. The only goal that you should vow to stick with is to not treat your body as if it is a fad, unworthy of longevity. Instead, work towards health and a healthy relationship between your mind, body, and spirit.

Chapter Nine

The Balanced Diet

Now we get into what so many fad diet supporters call the long running fad of nutrition. It is interesting to me, and somewhat alarming, that so many scientists and pseudoscientists have put in so much effort to debunk what has been established as truthfulness through many studies and across multiple generations of research. The body is dependent on a variety of nutrients, minerals, and vitamins that cannot be found in a single food group source but rather requires the intake of multiple food sources, often collectively, in order to ensure that the body is able to absorb and utilize these essential elements. No study, or none that I have encountered, has been able to debunk these studies but rather many studies have sought to find a 'work around' that would lead to optimal results (also known as media approved results) based on social standards of the time. Wait. I believe that we discussed these popularity trends at some point and referred to them as FADS! Every study and every attempt to alter the current knowledge about the needs of the body have been based on the concept that the role of the human body is to rapidly transform to meet the image standards of media content. Little, if any, attention has been given to the long term implications of these fads or to the sustainability of life, even the human race, should everyone comply with the standards presented by these pseudoscientists. Instead, the media continues to claim that there is some way to offset the needs of the body (needs that have been present since long before the media) in order to achieve a popularity that will fade faster than the temporary results promised. Now that I have spent a moment on my soapbox, I think we can get to the actual relevance of a balanced diet for optimal health and weight loss.

What is a balanced diet? I am certain that you have seen those poorly illustrated food pyramids since you were in early grade school and hoped that your plate would never look as unsavory! Fortunately, the U.S. Department of Agriculture has made the imagery far more appealing. The concept is simple. Our bodies need fruits and vegetables for essential nutrients and vitamins including fiber to ensure proper digestion. Any fad diet that limits the intake of this food group significantly hinders overall health and places the dieter at risk for any number of negative health implications. The U.S. Department of Agriculture explains that eating fruits and vegetables does not have to be costly when seasonal options are utilized. In brief, it is important to remember that nature will provide what is necessary. If a certain fruit or vegetable is in season, it is more affordable and packed with the nutrients that are necessary for health. Of course, it is important to also recognize that nature is a colorful lady. By balancing the colors of the fruits and vegetables, it is possible to ensure that all your nutritional needs are being met. Besides, how much more enjoyable is a colorful plate of food? Granted, plant options are not enough to sustain the body. The U.S. Department of Agriculture states that you should make at least half of your grain options whole grains. For weight loss, a higher percentage is recommended. For your protein intake, the U.S. Department of Agriculture recommends a variety to ensure that you are taking in all the possible benefits. Finally, the U.S. Department of Agriculture recommends that dairy products be selected in the lowest fat content.

Wait, so the U.S. Department of Agriculture is suggesting that all food groups can be safely and moderately consumed in such a way as to ensure that all nutrients, minerals, and vitamins are provided to the body without excessive fat or sugar intake and without concerns of dehydration and deficiencies? Certainly, such an approach must lead to excessive weight gain. After all, this means giving in to everything that the body needs. What kind of relationship are we trying to establish? The bottom line is this. The body needs what it needs because its job is to sustain YOU. Your job, then, is to sustain the body by ensuring that it has what it needs. The problem is that the balance between the food groups is often too difficult to integrate when the options are in front of you. I do not know about you, but my biggest concern has always been whether I will feel full or satisfied leaving the table. The fad diets offer ways to curb the appetite but they do not offer these options in such a way as to promote optimal health. But I want to feel full, healthy, and lose weight! Consider the lowest calorie options first. Your fruits and vegetables should take up a large portion of your plate followed by healthy, whole grains that will provide long term appetite suppression. Dairy products and protein should complete your meal. Based on your caloric needs at your current weight versus your goal weight, a gradual shift in intake should take place. There is no need for shifting your body into a state of starvation. Focus on healthy, filling calories and leave out the calories void of nutritional value. Really, you do not have to omit food groups. You simply have to consider your goals and realize that this is a marathon and not a sprint. That is, of course, unless we are back to considering this journey and your body as a fad!

CHAPTER TEN

EXERCISE

I am now going to use those two little four letter words that we all hate to talk about when we are seeking a quick fix for weight loss. EXER… CISE… That's right! I said it. Now, let's combine these profanities and get down to business. Exercise does not have to be scary. I repeat. Exercise does not have to be scary. Yet, just because it does not HAVE to be does not mean that it is not. I mean, really, have you seen these advertisements for the extreme workouts and the price tags on these pieces of equipment that promise unbelievable results? Have you watched the pounds literally drop off of these men and women during the hour long informercials? Yes. I have seen it all but might I remind you of the empty promises of the fad diets? Can I bring you back to the reality that health is about more than shedding pounds in front of a media outlet? Do you really believe that the results that are shown are the true results? I did not think so. Now that we have made it through that discussion, we can get to the nitty gritty of exercise.

How much do you currently exercise? An hour jog? Strenuous weight lifting? Dancing while house cleaning? Managing to walk to the mailbox each day? Regardless of your answer…good for you! Seriously, we do not give ourselves enough credit for the things that we do in a day. If we did, then we could see where we could do just a little bit more. Full disclosure, I do not jog an hour a day. Who has time for that? I enjoy dancing around with those 2lb dumbbells you can grab at Walmart for a few dollars but I cannot say that I do this every day. However, I am going to give myself credit because I do integrate as much as I think that I can. Comically, as I give myself credit, I realize that maybe, just maybe, I could have danced a few more moments. Maybe, when I went to check the mail, I could have taken a quick stroll around the block. Perhaps, when I was loading the dishwasher, I could have made one more trip around the house to look for glasses that were left sitting on end tables or nightstands. Can I do more? Certainly! Can you? Exercise does not necessarily mean making a one year commitment to a fitness club that you will later forget to cancel and end up paying for years later. It does not have to mean buying new equipment or comparing your results to those of others. Exercise is increasing your physical activity from what you are now doing to a greater intensity or frequency.

Shhh. Do not tell anyone that I just admitted that. I mean, after all, am I not supposed to write health books that help to promote the health industry? Should I not tell you that buying equipment and placing it in your home will motivate you to be more active? Join a team and pay membership dues. Buy an exercise bike and extend your closet. Above all, pay your due respect to all of those who have worked so hard to bring you fad diets so that the exercise industry can really feel the effects. Okay. But seriously. I am not here to promote anything or anyone but you. You are the only one who knows if you carry your laundry down the stairs or if you take the elevator. You are the only one who knows if you take the first available parking spot or if you drive in circles for hours to get as close to the door as humanly possible. You know how much you are putting in. I am here to ask you how much you expect to get out. Simply put, exercise is the process of increasing your use of calories. As a balanced diet is intended to control that intake to the point of supporting your current caloric needs, the purpose of exercise is to expend more calories than is consumed.

So, if that late night infomercial speaks to you and you believe that you will use that equipment, I support your decision. However, if that purchase will prevent you from being able to balance your diet this week, then I ask that you reconsider. There are many opportunities to increase your physical activity level. Just as your diet does not need a fad, neither does your exercise regimen. You simply need to commit, not to a fad diet, but to your health. You are what matters. You and your relationship with your body will determine your sustainability. You and your relationship with your diet and exercise will determine your weight loss journey. After all, there is nothing short live about your desire to want to live your best life. So I guess exercise is not the collectiveness of two four letter words but rather the collective decision to simply do a bit more today than was done yesterday.

CHAPTER ELEVEN

SLEEP HABITS

I do not know about you, but all of that talk about exercise sure made me tired. You know, that is the point. If we eat right and exercise, then our bodies will naturally be tired when it is time to sleep. So, wait, does this mean that a healthy diet and adequate exercise will improve your sleep. Yes, it does. But what does this have to do with a healthy weight loss? The fact is that adequate sleep will actually help to regulate your metabolic systems to ensure proper utilization of your caloric intake (Chaput & Tremblay, 2012). In other words, when your body systems are given adequate rest (ie you actually go to bed at night) then they are better prepared to fulfill their duties to your body and your overall health. In fact, according to Chaput and Tremblay (2012) there is a growing body of research that shows that inadequate sleep, often due to the rigorous requirements placed on people in today's technological and economical driven society, is directly related to the social trend of obesity that has increased the burden of healthcare for all members of society. In other words, the research shows that inadequate sleep contributes to obesity. As such, it is easy to defer that an adequate amount of sleep will lead to weight loss.

But wait, modern society supports a lifestyle that does not support adequate sleep. This means that a lack of sleep is popular and therefore, a fad. Yes! Pushing yourself to burning the candle at both ends will result in negative health outcomes. In this case, it will result in unhealthy weight gain and all of the known and unknown comorbidities associated with being overweight. However, a healthy diet and exercise are known to lead to better sleep and therefore, beyond their obvious benefits to weight loss, can indirectly contribute to this factor. To be clear, a body that is well rested is able to counter the negative implications of modern diet which has been confirmed across countless studies inclusive of participants that were not involved in fad diets. Simply getting adequate sleep has been shown as a proven method to prevent weight gain and promote overall healthy weight loss. As an added benefit, other avenues of weight loss including a healthy balanced diet and an increase in physical activity, no matter how small of an increase, have been shown to promote better sleep patterns.

What is the relationship between energy intake and output when considering adequate sleep? This has been the topic of inquiry for countless studies. In fact, to Chaput and Tremblay (2012) explained that the results of these studies have shown that those who do not get enough sleep are prone to the body's natural response of conserving energy in the form of calorie storage. In other words, the body, once again, responds to the negligence of the individual to provide it with what it actually needs by storing energy or mass against the individual's wishes. In other words, the body will make sure that it is sustainable until the point that no balance can be achieved. This means that restoring a balance or realizing the importance of this relationship will greatly reflect your own sustainability. Are you a fad or are you sustainable? The answer lies in your ability to give in to what your body needs. In this scenario, it is sleep. While this is supported by all other scenarios, it is reiterated, again, that one cannot be dismissed for the benefit of the other. The human body, and the human experience, are intertwined to such a point as one cannot exist without the other. Eat right and exercise but also make certain that your body has time to prepare for the long run.

CHAPTER TWELVE

SOCIAL SUPPORT

So, I have spent the majority of this book telling you that weight loss and health are not a popularity contest but rather are a person pursuit dependent on your inner relationships between your mind, body, and spirit. Now, I must tell you that this does not mean that you are alone in your journey and you should not pursue this goal alone. Can you? Certainly, many people have taken on life changes on their own and made great strides in personal development. It is absolutely possible and if you find yourself without a social support team, then know that you are not alone but that I am in your corner cheering you on. But from a serious outlook on life changes, most people have others who participate in their day to day routines. Do you eat with family? Coworkers? Do you meal share at the office or plan your grocery shopping with your significant other? Do your children require a certain snack cabinet that you swear off from but find yourself raiding in the middle of the night when life is finally quiet? It would be simplistic, almost easier, to state that no one is responsible for your eating habits than yourself. Of course, in the real world, we can blame a swarm of others. Now, we can stop there (blame is fun and empowering) or we can admit to ourselves that we allow this and want better. We can assume that those in our lives also want better for us. Now, we have to ask them. I know the fear. What if they do not want to change? What if they actually state that this is a "me" problem? They are right. It is a "me" problem, but we are a we. Now, my problem is a we problem and I am asking if they will help me fix it.

Does this mean that I am suggesting that you leave your significant other because they still want fried chicken on Monday nights? Of course not. I am, however, suggesting that you prepare yourself a grilled chicken breast and you ask that they make either positive or no comments about your choice. I am then suggesting that you find like minded friends. Find someone who will walk around the block or someone to call when those late night snack cravings set in. There is nothing wrong with you stating that you need a change. You are making a choice to be in this for the long haul. You are making a commitment, not to a fad diet, but to your loved ones, that you are going to overcome the barriers of weight and become a more active participant in life. You are asserting that you are not a fad.

Okay, now that I have given way too much insight into my own personal conflicts with seeking a social support structure, I can now give you information about what has eventually worked. There was never this great epitome moment when everyone who loved me said that they would immediately change every tradition in order to help me achieve my weight loss and health goals. There was no consensus among my friends that led to the end of Taco Tuesdays or the shift from Saturday movies to Saturday nights at the gym. Instead, I had to decide, for myself, that I could decide which activities that I would participate in and which activities I would pursue on my own. Scary, I know. But do you know what happened? I did not lose a single friend but, instead, I gained an entire new group of friends. On Taco Tuesdays, I had a taco salad and left (most) of the deep fried shell. On Saturdays, I went to the gym with my new friends and then met up with my old friends after the movie. I got the best spoilers unless I threw a fit preventing them from saying a word. Everyone could see that I was gaining a new set of confidence. Everyone could see that I was in it for the long haul.

Change is scary. Trust me, I know. But it is also beautiful and freeing. I thought that if I redirected my focus towards myself, then everyone would think that I was being selfish. I thought that if I changed my interests, then everyone that shared my interests would no longer be there. But here is the funny thing, I am not a fad and neither are you. The people who love you will support you. This does not mean that they will all sweat it out with you at the gym. This is not everyone's pursuit. This is yours. Social support does not mean that everyone changes with you but rather that everyone that matters supports your changes. Hopefully, you will be able to inspire those that you love to make positive changes in their own lives. If not, however, do not perceive their journeys as a hindrance to your own. Social support is important but how you perceive the support is important to your journey. I am here for you. Believe in the support but, when it becomes evident that it is not there, do not feel guilty about supporting your own sustainability.

CHAPTER THIRTEEN

MENTAL HEALTH

There cannot be a discussion of overall health without also discussing the complexities of mental health. I have included a very brief overview of eating disorders but I must ask you a simple question. Why are you seeking weight loss? I applaud you for landing on a book that focuses on healthy weight loss and I am more than proud of your emphasis on overall health which is evident at this point of your reading consistency. However, I wonder if you have given adequate consideration as to the relationship between weight loss, health and mental health. Firstly, let me override all the stigmatizations that are present when someone mentions mental health because I certainly do not mean to alarm you. In no way am I insinuating that a desire to lose weight indicates some form of mental illness. Mental illness and mental health are not interchangeable concepts. Mental illness, which also should not be stigmatized, is characterized by a neurological response. Mental health refers to how you perceive yourself and your relationship with others. Is this pursuit in response to a health concern, a diagnosis, or a legitimate consideration of your body mass index or are you responding to a media image or the expectations of someone in your life? Are you aware of the healthy weight for your body type or are you seeking to lose weight based on what you believe you should be? Mental health is not a diagnosis but rather a true concern for understanding why someone is exhibiting certain behaviors.

When I decided to include a discussion of mental health in the overall presentation of a healthy weight loss, I realized that the relationship between overall health and a healthy weight is not as obvious to some as it is to others. This is not a statement of health literacy but a clear assertion as to how many people view mental health as a secondary factor rather than a contributing factor. I remember as an adolescent, feeling the pressures of academic success and the demands of a clear course from high school to higher education to career, I began to feel a sense of loss. When I expressed this to my father, he explained that a teenager does not know the meaning of depression. Granted, I grew up in a loving home and in no way was my father dismissive of my needs. However, the very mention of a term associated with mental health set off a generational stigmatization that meant I could not seek help for this feeling. Now that I am older, I realize that mental health is directly linked to overall health and that a feeling of depression or isolation can quickly lead to weight gain or other unhealthy behaviors that can have long term negative implications. Again, I focus your attention on overall health. This is different from achieving an ideal weight but not dismissive of the pursuit of a healthy weight. You are a beautiful human who should be focused on the long run. However, it is important that this is not only a physical pursuit. Are you happy? Is your weight loss journey intended to add to your happiness and longevity or to replace a deficit that should otherwise be addressed?

You did not gain weight due to a single factor. You did not become the you that you are today without interactions with others. You are the collectiveness of your life experiences and it is time that you become more aware as to how these experiences have shaped your emphasis on our health. Although my father meant me no harm when he questioned my stance, it shaped my perception of my mental health. I believed for the longest time that mental health was separate from physical health and, as long as I could secure my physical health, I could consider myself sustainable. However, mental health leads to unhealthy behaviors, including an unhealthy relationship with food, that can negatively affect our ability to positively pursue longevity. Therefore, when you come to me, either directly or through reading the words that I type in the present, and ask me how to achieve a healthy weight loss that is sustainable and that will promote a healthy and long life, I cannot comprehensively answer that question without suggesting that you ensure that your mental health is sound. If not, seek help. Tell people who love you even if their answer may not meet your expectations. Find strength in their questions and seek answers on your own. You cannot pursue life changes unless you know your psychological reasons for these changes. At the very least, without such an understanding, these changes will not be sustainable.

CHAPTER FOURTEEN

SPIRITUAL HEALTH

I have been torn on whether or not to include this section in a book focused on weight loss but I have found myself drawn to your pursuit for an overall sense of health as has been reflected in the mere fact that you have not stopped your participation when I debunked many of the get thin quick fad diets that are most often the focus of internet searches about weight loss. I have openly questioned why so many pseudoscientists and fad diet enthusiasts have actively engaged in sharing stories that do not reflect long term data. I have acknowledged that many people only seek the short term results and I have tried in all of my capacity to not seem judgmental of these pursuits. I have given way to the evidence, what little has been present, and even identified my own areas of biasness. Yet, through it all, I have maintained that my goal is not to see you meet some media image of popularity but rather to walk you through your own journey of achieving a healthy weight that will promote your own sense of overall health. As such, I cannot justify a close to this discussion without also including the relevance of your spiritual health in this pursuit. Before I begin this discussion, please not that spiritual health is different from religious ideology and I, in no way, intend to reflect my personal beliefs as being relevant to your own pursuit of overall health. I do, however, intend to reflect the relationship between the acknowledgement of longevity, the importance of health, and the meaning of life as felt through spiritual health as a means to support and, to some extent, justify your personal pursuit toward weight loss and overall health.

While the literature is limited, perhaps due to concerns such as my own in addressing this connectivity, there has been research that shows a direct relationship between comfort eating and spiritual health. Specifically, Hawk, Goudy, and Gast (2003) found that individuals with a lesser emphasis on spiritual health report a higher occurrence rate of comfort eating to fill a void that is indescribable or unidentified. In other words, regardless of the form of religious ideology, a spiritual belief takes on the form of filling a void that could otherwise be filled with caloric intake or other unhealthy behaviors. In fact, Hawk, Goudy, and Gast (2003) "Responding to emotional states without turning to food may be a key skill required by some individuals to achieve and maintain weight loss. The possible role of such psychosocial constructs as self-esteem and spiritual well-being in mediating this process is intriguing" (pg. 33). In other words, there is a direct relationship between turning to foods, emotional regulation, and spiritual health that can no longer go unrecognized in our pursuit for an understanding of overall health. Does it matter what your spiritual beliefs are? Absolutely not. What matters is that you have a fulfilling relationship with your spiritual health that does not interfere but rather supports your relationship with your physical self.

This now leads to the actualization of understanding what spiritual health means to weight loss. After all, you sought this book as a means to healthy weight loss and here I have focused on your overall health. I have given you several examples as to how to not be healthy and then told you that weight loss is only a part of an overall pursuit of health. Guess what. I am not changing this stance. But I will make the connection more evident. In the beginning of this book, I told you that you are not a fad, your body is not a fad, and your pursuit for weight loss is not a fad. I told you that you have a purpose to fulfill based on your ability to pursue health and longevity in the mortal sense that should not be hindered by any other individual or consideration. Your health is your stance in the present and anything that prevents your longevity is a hinderance to your purpose. Do you see where I am going? Your spiritual health defines your purpose. It helps you define why you must beat the odds of longevity. Why are you trying to lose weight? Not because of a fad but because you have a greater purpose. Not because you know that purpose without a doubt but because you have faith that this purpose will manifest. Your spiritual health has everything to do with who you are and what you will become. Do not dismiss it in the pursuit of your physical health.

Chapter Fifteen

Towards a Healthy Balance

We have now reached the point that we can no longer talk abstractly about what is expected of you if you expect to achieve a healthy weight while avoiding the pitfalls of fads and asserting your claim to longevity despite any challenges or barriers that you have realized in your life. I have sugar coated this journey to the point that one might question my own ability to forgo sweets in the pursuit of happiness and health. I have laid out every possible excuse, every alternative diet plan, and every reason for not pursuing your journey towards health. I have given you an array of reasons why this plan or that plan will not work and even questioned your motivation. Still yet, you are still here with me. You are wondering what I will say next. You are looking for my next avenue of justification that will allow you to go on about your normal lifestyle under the pretense that you are protecting your mental health, spiritual health, or social circle. You are now expecting that I would answer my phone in the middle of the night and tell you that it is okay to eat comfort foods with your significant other if that makes you feel a sense of happiness and, by some oddity, health. However, I will not answer that call and, if I did, it would be filled with so many questions that only you can answer.

What is your goal? Where do you see yourself in five or ten years? Are you still here in twenty or even fifty years? If you are not here, to what spiritual entity are you explaining your life's course? Are you happy with your decisions? I am not here to judge you. I do not have a direct answer as to what it means to be healthy. I know that you came here wondering how to lose weight and I have told you that there is no quick answer to this question. I have given you the science as to why you must look at your whole health in order to achieve a healthy weight and why every decision is relevant. I have been understanding with the realization that the concept of exercise is as media influenced as the concept of the perfect body image. However, I have also been upfront with how easy it is to gradually increase your physical activity. You did not get to the point of searching for and reading this book in a single moment nor will you achieve your health goals in such brevity. Instead, we are on this journey together. I am proud of the steps that you have taken to this point. But I ask that you do not stop now. I ask that you consider your whole health and the implications to yourself, your loved ones, and the larger society.

As such, I ask that you begin the transition towards a healthy balance. Health is not achieved through the acknowledgement of fad diets. It is not achieved through identifying with the popularity contests that are dependent on the media's betrayal of what is the perfect body image. Health is achieved through a balance that has long been lost in the emphasis of the media. What is healthy to you? Do you need to follow some trend of popularity to be healthy? If so, are your prepared both mentally and spiritually to respond to the negative implications of this pursuit? Our bodies are not immortal even if there is an indication that ourselves, through spirituality may be. Yet, in all of my studies of religious ideologies, I have not found a single belief set that supports hinderances to physical health as a means to achieving spiritual health. In other words, there is not doctrine that supports the dismissal of the mind and body in support of the spiritual self. Instead, there is consistent support for achieving a balance that can only be defined as whole health. It is that form of health that I wish for you.

CHAPTER SIXTEEN

CONCLUSION

When I began writing this book, or even more transparent, when I began considering writing this book, I was not certain what information should be included. I knew that I had watched many friends fall victim to the popular fad diets only to experience significant weight gain when the diets were not sustainable and the resulting mental health concerns associated with yo yo dieting. The only thing that kept me motivated was not the commonalities between my friends but rather the realization that others beyond my social circle, might be experiencing the same scenarios without the social support that we have all been afforded. Granted, I do not mean to dismiss our plight because we have been blessed with support no more than I would expect that you would want your own to be left out of the discussion. We all struggle with who we are and who we are supposed to be and, quite frankly, that is okay. What is not okay, however, is that we so often feel the need to give in to circumstances and social norms that we forget that we are so much more than that. This is why I have written this book.

I do not know you, or maybe I do. I have not experienced life in the same way that you have or maybe, to some extent, I have. I may never meet you in real life or maybe we will share a table at a diner in some not so distant future. Regardless, we are in this together. This life that is before us is ours to change, mold and alter as we see fit. But our contributions end when we decide to no longer participate. We begin to fade away when we accept that we are nothing more than fads. We give up our right to longevity when we pursue avenues that do not support our sustainability. I understand the drive to fit in and the belief that who we are is defined by who accepts us. I get that it is a common belief that fitting the perfect mold means being perfect if only for a moment. I promise you, I get it. However, we are a smart species. We are able to decipher evidence, ensure our longevity, and create a world greater than nature intended. Are we really that susceptible to fads?

I started this journey to write a book focused on weight loss but I felt more compelled to write about how weight loss is perceived in the journey for overall health. Have we, as a society, forgotten the importance of whole health? Certainly, I support your journey in achieving a healthy weight goal and I hope that you achieve this goal not through a fad diet but rather through a focus on a balanced diet, exercise, mental, and spiritual health. I believe, based on extensive research, that this will help you not only to achieve your weight loss goals but also to sustain these goals as well as your overall health. We, as a society, must be supportive in one another's pursuits of health even when these pursuits do not reflect the popular notions. We must support these pursuits of health even when the stigmatizations of mental health and the diversification of spiritual health means accepting one another. But most importantly, regardless of the fads and despite all of the media portrayals, you have a responsibility to yourself and others to live your best and healthiest life. After all, your body is not a fad, and neither are you.

REFERENCES

Ellenbroek, J. H., van Dijck, L., Töns, H. A., Rabelink, T. J., Carlotti, F., Ballieux, B. E., & de Koning, E. J. (2014). Long-term ketogenic diet causes glucose intolerance and reduced β-and α-cell mass but no weight loss in mice. *American Journal of Physiology-Endocrinology and Metabolism, 306*(5), E552-E558.

Chaput, J. P., & Tremblay, A. (2012). Adequate sleep to improve the treatment of obesity. *Cmaj, 184*(18), 1975-1976.

Hawks, S. R., Goudy, M. B., & Gast, J. A. (2003). Emotional eating and spiritual well-being: A possible connection?. *American Journal of Health Education, 34*(1), 30-33.

Heaner, M. (2013). Detox Diets: myths vs. reality. *IDEA Fitness Journal, 10*(2), 58-61.

Khawandanah, J., & Tewfik, I. (2016). Fad diets: Lifestyle promises and health challenges. *Journal of Food Research, 5*(6), 80.

Mamounis, K. J. (2017). The Dangers of Fat Metabolism and PUFA: Why You Don't Want to be a Fat Burner. *Journal of Evolution and Health, 2*(1), 9.

Pilis, W., Stec, K., Zych, M., & Pilis, A. (2014). Health benefits and risk associated with adopting a vegetarian diet. *Roczniki Państwowego*